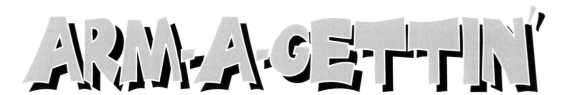

# Your Guide to Building Massive Arms

## By Robert Kennedy

This book is not intended as medical
advice, nor is it offered for use in the
diagnosis of any health condition or as
a substitute for medical treatment
and/or counsel. Its purpose is to explore
advanced topics on sports nutrition and
exercise. All data is for information only.
Use of any of the programs within this
book is at the sole risk and choice of
the reader.

Copyright ©2002 by Robert Kennedy

Published by MuscleMag International
5775 McLaughlin Road
Mississauga, ON
Canada L5R 3P7

Designed by Jackie Thibeault
Edited by Sandy Wheeler

National Library of Canada cataloguing in publication

Kennedy, Robert, 1938
    Arm-a-gettin': your guide to building massive arms/ by Robert Kennedy

Includes bibliographical references.
ISBN 1-55210-027-8

    1. Bodybuilding. 2. Arm exercises. I. Title.

GV546.5.K443 2002     646.7'5     C2002-905490-7


Distributed in Canada by
CANBOOK Distribution Services
1220 Nicholson Road
Newmarket, ON
Canada L3Y 7V1

Distributed in the United States by
BookWorld Services
1933 Whitfield Park Loop
Sarasota, FL 34243

Printed in Canada

# Table of Contents

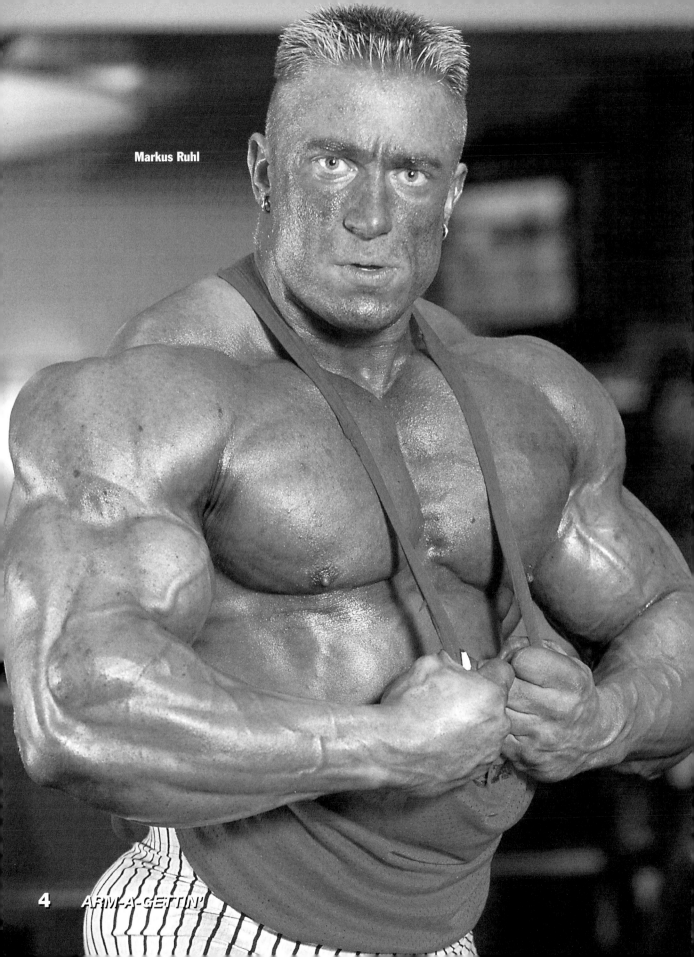

Markus Ruhl

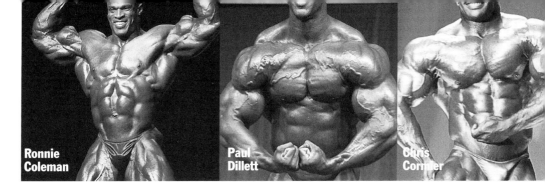

Ronnie Coleman

Paul Dillett

Chris Cormier

# Introduction

There's nothing like a hot pair of arms. Yes, a well-built chest is fine, and muscular legs are nice, but the real aim of almost every guy who trains is to build a pair of powerful, muscular, *big arms*. For some intangible reason the arms create a special effect in the appearance of the male physique, and the more muscular the appearance the better. You can add size to that definition of muscular arms as well. A nasty pair of arms is what you might consider as *"prime beef"* – the best of the best, big and full of muscle.

Would you consider your arms as *prime beef?* Or perhaps they fall short. Although most guys would like to have a pair of big and cut arms, few actually do. Wishing won't do the trick – it is training that builds those arms into monsters of size and muscularity. This book will provide you with training programs, tips and techniques for building your own pair much bigger than they currently are. You can use these training programs to stimulate new muscle growth in your arms. And you can put the training tips and insight to work as well in promoting more muscle mass in the upper arm region. The sooner you get going the better – so start down the path to arm mass today.

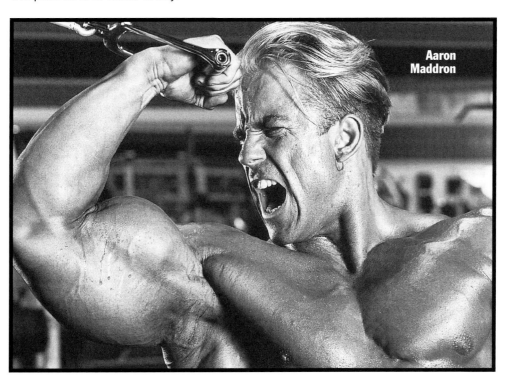

Aaron Maddron

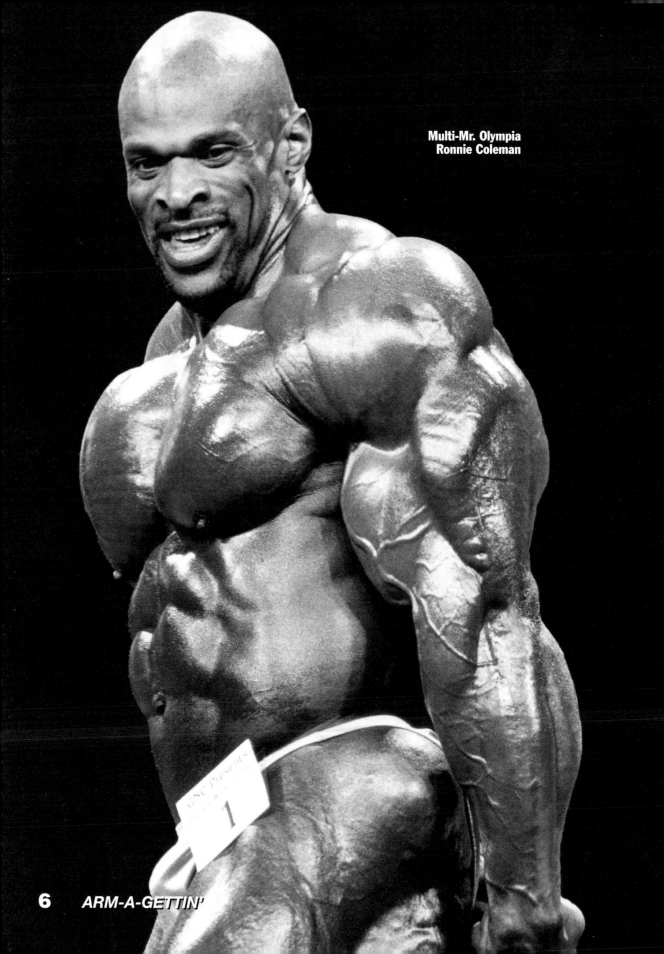

Multi-Mr. Olympia
Ronnie Coleman

*ARM-A-GETTIN'*

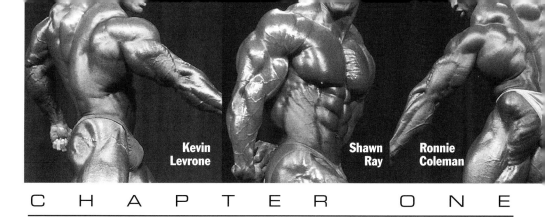

Kevin Levrone

Shawn Ray

Ronnie Coleman

*Triceps?* You wanted to start with the biceps, right? Building that mountain of muscle on top of the arm is enticing, and many guys get caught up in the "biceps first" approach. In fact that is one of the most certain signs of being a novice – spending most of your arm-training time, and even most of your overall training time, on the biceps. This stumbling block is hard to overcome. However, triceps provide the essential muscle base to building massive arms. Here's why: The triceps comprise more muscle mass than do the biceps.

# Triceps Routines

The biceps, when trained, put a nice mound of muscle on top of the bone of the upper arm. The triceps, however, put a huge group of mounds underneath the bone of the upper arm. The triceps contains more body mass area, and it is wise to prioritize your triceps-training if you want big arms. The name of each muscle group gives away which contains the most major muscles – *bi* is two muscles, *tri* is three muscles. And the breakdown between the two looks roughly like this for upper-arm mass: triceps = 66 percent of upper-arm muscle area, biceps = 34 percent of the upper-arm muscle area. If you want to push the tape measure out an inch or two more, it is essential to camp out in the triceps-training area. Why?

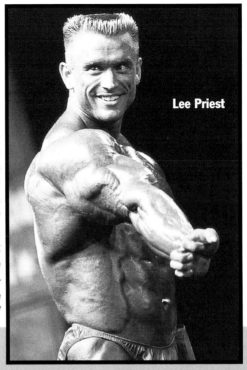

**Lee Priest**

Simply because big triceps equates to big arms. This fact may shock you if you have been working your biceps super-hard during your workout career, but it is true. And the reason you don't have the arm size you want may be that you haven't been putting enough emphasis into the triceps-training. This is not to say the biceps are not important – they are. But the triceps are *more important.* Get it through your head now and you will save yourself a lot of training time and effort – the triceps are more important than the biceps in the overall arm size/shape/muscularity scheme.

Yes, the triceps are more crucial to upper-arm size and shape than the biceps, and knowing that should give you a strong incentive to prioritize your

**Prioritize your triceps-training if you want truly big arms.**

training to make the triceps workout of chief importance. If you must skip one of your arm workouts, make it biceps rather than a triceps workout. Learn it again and again – triceps are *numero uno* for the arms. Plan on spending quite a bit of energy to build some mass into your triceps.

The triceps muscles get involved as a primary muscle group when a pushing motion occurs. The triceps are the main impetus in moving an object away from the body when the arms are involved. Since many workouts involve the arms in pushing motions, you must set up the various workouts correctly so you do not overtax the triceps region, but you also mustn't understimulate them either.

The triceps heads can be worked with a variety of movements. Some more directly involve the upper and outer heads, others mainly hit the low end of the long triceps muscle. You're best to incorporate a strong mix of triceps stimulation in your training schedule and you will accomplish exactly that with the diverse group of triceps exercises presented here. The mechanics of the moves are explained so you can get started on overhauling your arm program right away. Often a slight variation in the exercise you are presently using will be the catalyst for new gains in muscle. Slight changes in the angle of the exercise, or a shift in the hand placement, can translate into strong changes in muscle stimulation. *Arm-a-Gettin'* will feature some tricks you may not have heard of before. Also included are a number of unique triceps specialty moves. These exercises can help you target your triceps for the renewal of growth in this region so vitally necessary for super arms.

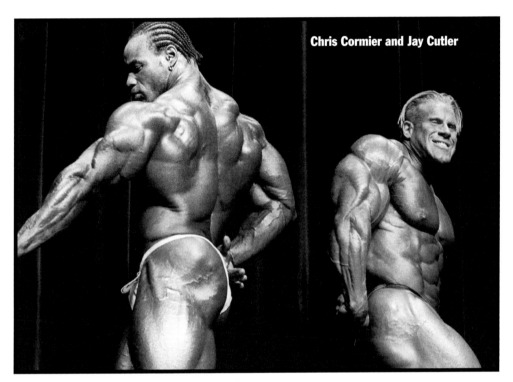
Chris Cormier and Jay Cutler

# Workout Schemes

The triceps muscles are involved in a variety of exercises. The way in which you schedule your overall *workout rotation* should influence your approach to triceps-training. There are two basic tracks. If your triceps-training is included with other exercises, especially pushing movements, you want to do fewer sets for triceps per workout. If your triceps-training is performed by itself, you want to do more triceps work. For example, if you are employing a push/pull split rotation, you would do less direct triceps-training because the triceps will be receiving a lot of work from the other pushing exercises.

**The triceps are more important than the biceps for building arm size and shape!**

The overhead press and dumbell press as used in shoulder-training both strongly involve the triceps. The bench press and dumbell press in chest-training both strongly involve the triceps. If you perform your triceps-training the

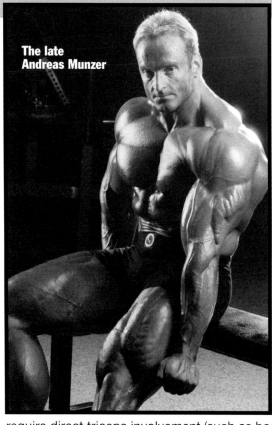

The late Andreas Munzer

same day as you work chest and shoulders, the best approach is to make the triceps-training *less involved.* For example, you may perform 3 or 4 sets of barbell presses, 3 or 4 sets of dumbell presses, 3 or 4 sets of bench presses, and 3 or 4 sets of incline barbell or dumbell presses in the course of the workout. All tolled, you may have pushed out 16 sets that require the triceps to lift the iron before you ever get to the specific triceps-training itself. At this point just a few sets of direct work, taking the triceps to a pumped state as fast as possible, will do the trick.

Another possibility is to work the triceps with one other bodypart, perhaps something that does not require direct triceps involvement (such as back or legs). You would be able to perform more sets for the triceps safely, without overtaxing the region. In the final scenario you devote the entire training session to triceps-training alone. In this case you can use more sets for direct triceps stimulation than with any other approach.

You must consider the overall workout strategy you employ and the entire weekly rotation as you set up your routine. No mistake about it – if you want big arms, you must prioritize the triceps-training. Plan to maximize the triceps-training time. This may translate into devoting a full workout session to triceps, and doubling up on other muscle groups at other times in the week to allow for concentration on the triceps.

Another prioritization tool that can be utilized is to give an extra day of rest to the triceps. For example, you may take a day off after training shoulders before lifting again (any bodypart), but for the triceps you would take off two days – or more, depending upon your recovery abilities. The extra rest not only lets the triceps grow back fully, but also ensures that they will be *fresh and full of energy* for next time – a key factor for a hot workout.

# Yates Favorites

There are dozens of great triceps exercises and many will be noted here in a variety of exercise settings. Why not start with the favorite triceps exercises of Dorian Yates? This Olympian believes in the heavy-duty, brief approach to training. He works only a few exercises per bodypart and so it is vital that he pick the best of the best to amass significant size. He reveals the following wisdom:

"I'd say 99 percent of my triceps development came from doing two movements. I've tried every triceps exercise imaginable and the best two I've found for packing on serious beef are *cable pressdowns* and *lying EZ-curl extensions.*"

Dorian's top choice are favorites of many bodybuilders. Dorian points out that the EZ-curl bar puts the wrist in a more natural position (slightly angled instead of bent straight). So how about a workout featuring Dorian's duo?

**Workout A**

| | | |
|---|---|---|
| EZ-curl prone extensions | 3-4 sets | 6-10 reps |
| Cable pressdowns (pushdowns) | 3-4 sets | 6-10 reps |

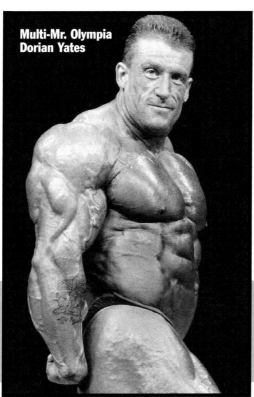

Multi-Mr. Olympia
Dorian Yates

As an advanced bodybuilder Dorian would use fewer sets. If you haven't quite arrived at his development you can afford to put in a few more sets than he would to fully stimulate your triceps. This workout would will well when the triceps-training is mixed in with other muscle groups. It is a wrap-up workout to bring out the pump in the triceps region. When you have more time to work the triceps alone, consider the same two exercises, but with more sets for each exercise for a full and concentrated blast on this vital region.

**The battle for the arms is won or lost with your triceps-training.**

**Workout B**

| | | |
|---|---|---|
| EZ-curl prone extensions | 5-6 sets | 6-10 reps |
| Cable pressdowns (pushdowns) | 5-6 sets | 6-10 reps |

Getting in more sets for each of the exercises works best when you are working the triceps on their own. You can also lighten up the set and use another triceps exercise that Dorian gives favorable mention – *the triceps dip.* And in order to bring out the mass, make it a *weighted dip.*

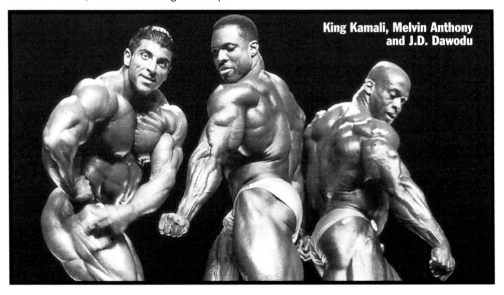

King Kamali, Melvin Anthony and J.D. Dawodu

**Workout C**

| | | |
|---|---|---|
| Weighted dips | 4 sets | 10 reps |
| EZ-curl prone extensions | 4 sets | 6-10 reps |
| Cable pressdowns (pushdowns) | 4 sets | 6-10 reps |

Workout C is a good 12-set blast at the triceps that will push them toward more size. You can also achieve a wonderful pump session by *supersetting* Dorian's two favorite exercises, which is workout D.

**The triceps receive a lot of action in any of a variety of workouts for other muscle groups, particularly the shoulders and chest.**

**Workout D**

| | | |
|---|---|---|
| EZ-curl prone extensions | 3-4 sets | 6-10 reps |
| *Superset with ...* | | |
| Cable pressdown (pushdown) | 3-4 sets | 6-10 reps |

This superset will be quite challenging for the final couple of sets but will reward you with a monster pump.

When performing the EZ-curl prone extension, consider a training tip from another Mr. Olympia, *Arnold Schwarzenegger.* Arnold once pointed out that the prone extension can be made more efficient by not quite letting the arms square with the body. Instead, hold the arms slightly backward so that when the arms come to a full extension in the upward position, they cannot rest and they remain under tension. Another option for maintaining tension on the triceps is found in using a cable instead of an EZ-curl bar and performing the movement on an incline bench, which is triceps workout E.

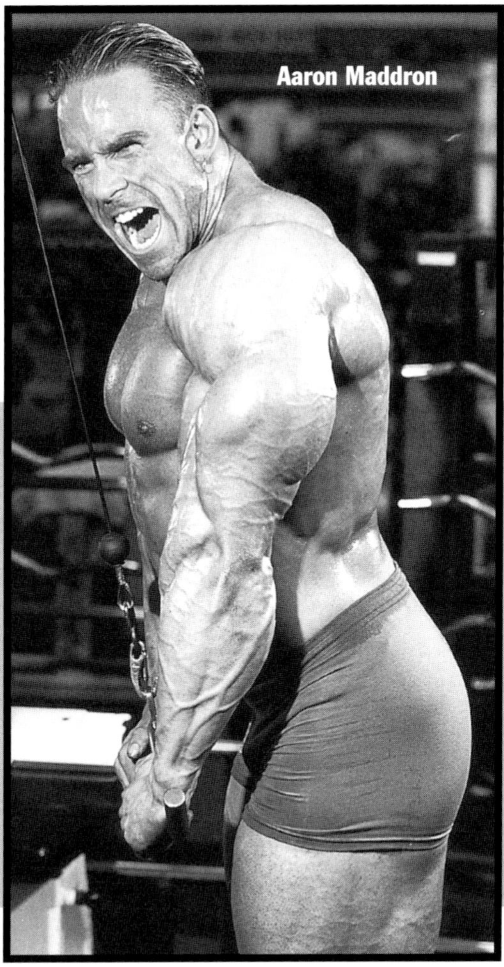

**Don't overload the triceps with a high-volume workout if you have also worked them via shoulder and chest-training earlier in the session.**

Aaron Maddron

**Workout E**

| | | |
|---|---|---|
| Incline cable extensions | 3-4 sets | 6-10 reps |
| Cable pressdowns (pushdowns) | 3-4 sets | 6-10 reps |

# The Magic of Constant Tension

For a musclebuilding variation, try using the extension movement on an incline with a cable. The incline angle, coupled with the pull of the weighted cable, keeps tension on the triceps throughout the full range of motion. The triceps receive no rest at the top of the move, and none elsewhere either as the weight on the cable keeps tugging at them. This constant tension adds up to more muscle stimulation and results in growth.

The incline cable extension is a great move that not too many people are aware of, but it will work wonders for packing more muscle into the triceps region. This move works on all three heads of the triceps, another good reason to try this unique exercise. If you have access to a cable pulley machine and a bench that inclines, make sure you add this exercise to your routine.

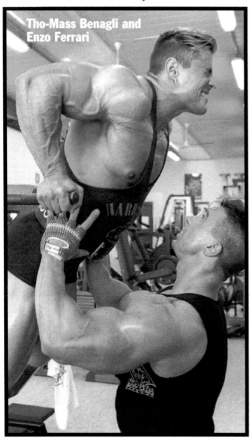

Tho-Mass Benagli and Enzo Ferrari

# Devastating Dip

The dip has been a favorite movement of the top pros for years. When used with a relatively narrow grip, it builds up incredible triceps. Add extra weight by strapping on a few more pounds to allow incrementally higher stress on the muscles. The weighted dip is a great exercise in itself. If you have used this exercise only in passing, now may be the time to give it serious consideration. Many point to the weighted dip as the best way to pack mass into the triceps. Another advantage is that it will really help to boost your poundages in the bench press. If you want a bigger bench, hit the dips hard and watch your poundages climb.

*Training Tip –* With the weighted dip it is always wise to perform the first set or so without weights. Get the elbows and chest warmed up for the full dip movement, and then start adding weight once you have gotten into the dipping groove. There are specially made weight belts that allow a plate or dumbell to be attached. Or you can make your own with a 3-4 inch nylon webbing belt, riveted together. Here is a workout for the triceps that features just the dip in multiple sets:

### Solo Dip Workout

| | | |
|---|---|---|
| Warmup: regular dips | 1-2 sets | 4-5 reps |
| Weighted dips | 8 sets | 8-10 reps |

### Reverse or Bench Dip

Regular dipping is not the only type that stimulates the triceps. The reverse dip – or bench dip – is another variation that can be employed with effective results. The bench dip is performed by placing your hands behind your glutes and on a bench. Support the rest of your body by placing your feet on a separate bench. At this point your body is the bridge between the two benches (both roughly the same height). Lower your body by bending your elbows, and then push up until your arms are fully extended. This pressing motion puts most of the emphasis on the tri-

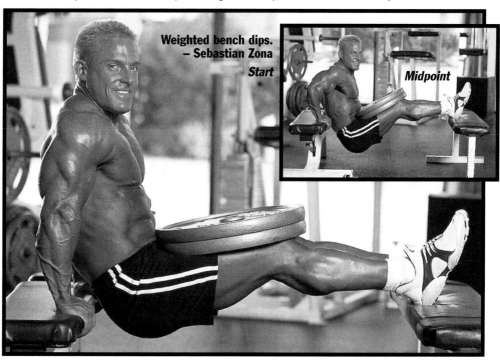

Weighted bench dips.
– Sebastian Zona

*Start*

*Midpoint*

ceps. The move can be made even more challenging in two ways. You can add resistance by putting a weight plate on your lap. You can also use a higher bench for your feet than the one for your hands. The bench dip is a wonderful all-round triceps exercise as it works all three heads of the triceps. For a real arm burn, try a mixture of the regular weighted dips superset with the bench dip.

**Superset Dip Workout**

| | | |
|---|---|---|
| Warmup: regular dips | 1-2 sets | 4-5 reps |
| Weighted dips | 4 sets | 8-10 reps |
| *Superset with …* | | |
| Bench dips, weighted | 4 sets | 10-12 reps |

# Pushdown/Pressdown Variations

The cable pushdown exercise, also called the pressdown by some people, can be performed in a variety of ways. With more than a few different styles of handles that

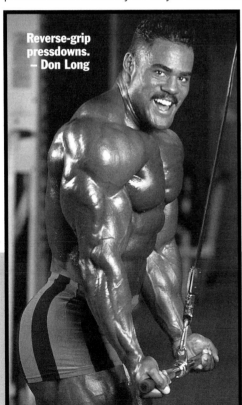

Reverse-grip pressdowns. – Don Long

can be attached to the cable pulley you can stimulate many different effects on the muscles being worked. The most standard attachment is the straight bar, which 90 percent of the people use to train their triceps. However, a simple twist of the wrist can make the exercise even more effective.

Reverse your grip on the bar and move from a palms-down position to a palms-up hand position. The exercise performed with this grip is the "reverse-grip pushdown" and it's a dandy. It works all three heads of the triceps and gives the entire region a fantastic burn. You will

**The more advanced you are, the fewer sets you need to stimulate the targeted muscles.**

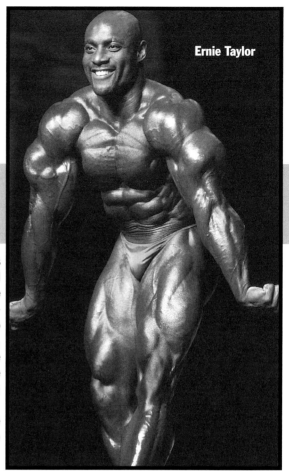

Ernie Taylor

## The cable press-down is also known as the pushdown.

need to begin with lighter weights but the move is more isolated and the lighter weights will work the muscle over hard. Many top professionals do the reverse-grip pressdown one arm at a time, alternating back and forth, one arm then the other. Some pros use a bent bar and push with both hands at once.

Here is a workout with the reverse-grip pressdown teamed up with the EZ-curl prone extension.

### Reverse-Grip Pressdown Workout

| | | |
|---|---|---|
| EZ-curl prone extensions | 4 sets | 8-10 reps |
| Reverse-grip cable pushdowns | 5 sets | 8-12 reps |

The single-arm reverse-grip cable pushdown allows for a great deal of concentrated effort directly on the three heads. This move works best at the end of a triceps routine when the muscles are already on fire from the previous training. Here is a single-hand reverse-grip workout:

### Reverse-Grip Pressdown Workout II

| | | |
|---|---|---|
| Weighted dips | 4 sets | 6-8 reps |
| One-arm reverse-grip cable pushdowns | 5 sets | 8-12 reps |

### Power Pushdown

The pushdown/pressdown move can be performed in a *power style* as well as a *finesse technique style.* Position the hands slightly wider than for regular pushdowns (out to a foot apart) and start with the bar up around the upper abdominal region. Bend forward ever so slightly, and push the bar down. You can load the plate stack up for this move after a couple of warmup sets to get the elbows loosened up.

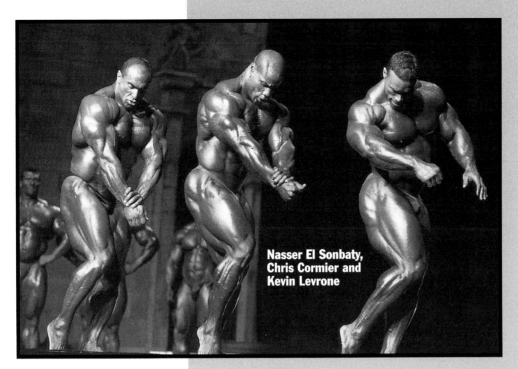

Nasser El Sonbaty,
Chris Cormier and
Kevin Levrone

## More Triceps Mass

**Triceps-training tip – Don't bring the bar up to a resting point in the upper position of the EZ-curl prone extension – instead, keep the arms slightly angled back for continuous tension.**

If you are still looking for massive triceps, here is another super exercise – the close-grip bench press, also termed the "triceps bench." This move is performed with the hands placed 6 to 12 inches apart, with the rest of the body in the same position as for the bench press. Bringing the arms in closer together takes most of the chest muscle involvement out of the action and puts the burden for moving the metal on the triceps.

The close-grip bench press allows for the use of very heavy weights and stimulates good size in the triceps. The best angle to take is to move the bar toward the high end of the chest as it goes up, and lower it down to middle or upper chest. Push the bar all the way up, but don't let it rest at the top or the bottom. Don't be tempted to let the bar sit on your chest even for a second in this exercise – it would take away the growth-producing tension.

Another slight variation is to place the hands out a little wider and go with the Gironda-style move of bringing the bar down closer to the neck region. The late Vince Gironda recommended a hand placement of roughly a foot apart, and bringing the bar down to the high upper chest region. Dr. Ollie McClay favors this high chest placement as well. Note – this is one of the few exercises where you can allow the elbows to flare out wide, as opposed to extension movements where you want to keep the elbows in as tight as possible.

When performing the standard close-grip bench press, put this hardcore exercise at the front end of the routine and use some heavy weights. Of course you want to start light in the beginning, but keep piling the weights on until you are handling some substantial iron in this power-enhancing musclebuilding exercise. And vary the repetitions within a wide range of 6 to 15 per set.

**Close-Grip Bench Workout**

| | | |
|---|---|---|
| Close-grip bench presses | 5 sets | 6-15 reps |
| Weighted dips | 1-2 sets | 10 reps |
| EZ-curl prone extensions | 3 sets | 10 reps |

You can work the close-grip bench press into any of a variety of training routines for a mass-stimulating effect.

Two- and three-exercise mixes are great for building the triceps, particularly when you work more than one muscle group in conjunction with the triceps-training. However, you can spread out to a greater number of exercises when you work the triceps alone or with another smaller muscle group like the biceps. Here is one such workout that starts off with the dip and moves on to an increasing number of sets for each exercise.

| | | |
|---|---|---|
| Dips, 1 warmup set | 1 heavy set | 5-10 reps |
| Close-grip bench presses | 2 sets | 10 reps |
| EZ-curl prone extensions | 3 sets | 8 reps |
| Reverse-cable pushdowns | 4 sets | 12 reps |

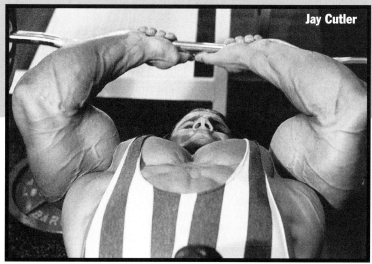

Jay Cutler

**Another name for the triceps extension exercise is the French press.**

Another very popular triceps exercise is the rope or V-bar pushdown on a cable pulley apparatus. Using these attachments will allow the hands to be in a more natural position than straight out. The moderate angle of the V-bar can also be achieved by using a rope attachment, and slightly angling the rope on the downstroke, with a wider angle at the bottom as the triceps are given a maximum contraction. The V-bar or rope pulley attachment works all three triceps heads and allows for a very deep muscle burn. If you train at home you might consider purchasing one of these attachments. They do not cost much and contribute quite a bit to a hot pair of arms.

**Workout Incorporating V-Bar and Rope Pushdown**

| | | |
|---|---|---|
| V-bar pushdowns | 4 sets | 10 reps |
| Close-grip bench presses | 3 sets | 8 reps |
| Rope pushdowns | 3 sets | 12-15 reps |

## Deep Stretch

One of the best things you can do to make sure you get good growth is to always focus on obtaining a good, deep stretch with each repetition, particularly in triceps extensions (prone, incline, etc.). A deep stretch helps you attain a full range of motion, and to even deepen that range over time as you push yourself a bit further. Hardcore training over the full range of motion adds up to bigger muscles. However, don't rush into a fully stretched out position initially – get there at a moderate pace, pushing a bit

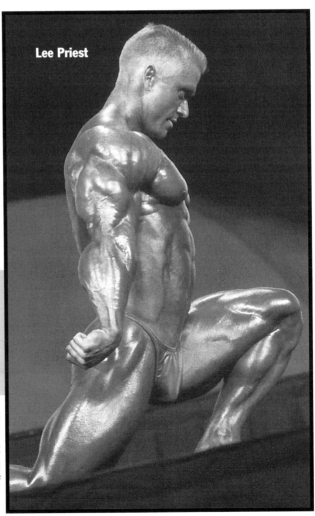

Lee Priest

**The incline cable French press keeps constant tension on the triceps.**

further each time out. Soon you will have a much broader range of motion and really get the muscles growing. Don't limit the range of your triceps-training too narrowly; go with a wider range of motion and build those muscles deep.

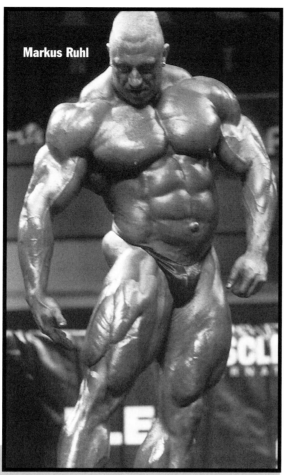

Markus Ruhl

# Super Musclebuilder

Everyone likes to find a super musclebuilder, one particular exercise that noticeably stimulates the muscles in an extreme manner. Some do so through experimentation on their own, others by trying something they have read about or seen someone else do in the gym. Here is a bona fide super musclebuilder – *the dumbell prone extension.*

This movement is performed similar to the EZ-curl prone extension. You lie face up on a bench and push the dumbells overhead in an extension motion. However, this exercise is even better than the EZ-curl version as it expands on the natural hand position and allows for more individual muscle control and flexibility. Top that off with even deeper concentration and you have one super exercise.

Grab a pair of light dumbells and lie prone, face up, on a bench. Hold the dumbells at arms' length overhead, and slowly lower them downward behind your head, using your elbow as a hinge. Keep the elbows pointed straight upward throughout the movement. Also keep the elbows as close to each other as possible. The wider you flare your elbows out to the sides, the less impact this movement (or any other) will have on the triceps. Keep them tight and close to your head at all times.

**Want to increase the poundage you use in the bench press? Start performing weighted dips and watch your bench press poundages rise as you increase the amount you dip with.**

There are not many key elements to good extension action, but the few that are essential must be followed – elbows in tight, elbows pointed straight up, and continuous tension on the triceps. Continuous tension in the dumbell prone extension is attained by not quite letting the arms straighten out over the body. Instead keep the arms at a slight angle to the body. Don't make the mistake of taking the weight only part of the way down – instead let the dumbells continue (in a controlled manner) back behind and below the head.

Any time weight is over the head is a good time to be cautious, so move the iron at a fairly slow pace. Use a light weight to learn how to get into the groove of this exercise, then go to heavier dumbells. Focus on maintaining good form. Force a good strong contraction at the top of the move, and a very deep stretch at the bottom. Once you do learn the working path for this exercise and start concentrating on your triceps throughout the movement, your arms should really take off. Total mental concentration during the dumbell prone extension is vital for the fullest muscle pump. Here is a workout featuring the dumbell prone extension:

| | | |
|---|---|---|
| Dips, weighted | 2 sets | 10 reps |
| Dumbell prone extensions | 4 sets | 8 reps |
| Reverse-grip pushdowns | 3 sets | 10-12 reps |

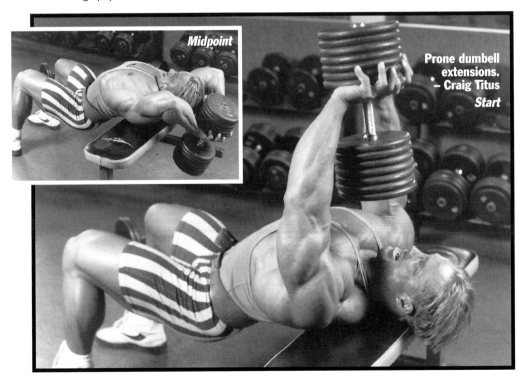

Midpoint

Prone dumbell extensions. – Craig Titus

Start

# Lower Triceps Thickness

Are your upper triceps looking fine but you need more fullness in the lower triceps area? Consider using the close-grip pushup, a good tool for attacking this often-neglected region. Ball your hands into a fist and put both fists on the floor, with the

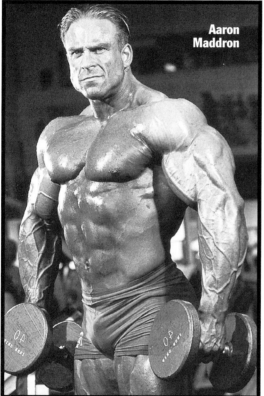

Aaron Maddron

back edge of the hand being the point that touches down. The hands should be about 6 inches apart. Perform this close-grip pushup for several sessions until you can pump out a high repetition count. Then you can make the exercise challenging again. Elevate your feet to put more pressure on the triceps and induce more growth. Once you master this position, you can then take it even one step further by adding resistance (in the form of a weighted vest for example) for maximum stimulation.

## Postworkout Triceps Pump

The triceps pump up fairly easily for most trainers during a workout, and usually the fire really gets going by the second exercise. You can promote the pump in the triceps area even further with what's called *the postworkout pump*. The postworkout pump is a deliberate movement aimed at provoking a massive pump in the upper arm area. This phase of the workout is after the last weighted set is finished (hence the name "post").

Place a bar across the bench press rack (or power rack) at roughly upper-abdomen height. Take a step or so back from the racked bar and lean forward, keeping the heels planted a couple of feet from the bar. Grasp the bar with a close-grip hand placement (6 to 8 inches apart) and push your body away from the bar, with heels remaining firmly in the same place. Lower your upper body back to the racked bar, and repeat. Use a high repetition range (15, 20 or even more) for a couple of sets

**The triceps pump at the end of a hard workout can significantly inflate the arms.**

to pump the triceps up like balloons. This move works very well as the triceps are already highly strung from the workout and a pump brings the effort together into a fantastic climax. A routine that includes the postworkout triceps pump looks something like this:

| | | |
|---|---|---|
| Close-grip bench presses | 3 sets | 8 reps |
| Dumbell prone extensions | 4 sets | 8 reps |
| V-bar pressdowns | 4 sets | 10 reps |
| Triceps pump on bar across bench press rack | 2 sets | 15+ reps per set |

For a high-voltage pump, try using the triceps pump at the end of each exercise and watch the backs of your arms blow up like balloons.

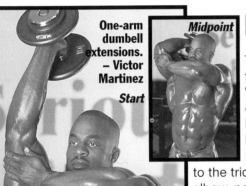

One-arm dumbell extensions. – Victor Martinez

*Start*

*Midpoint*

## Drawing the Sword

The one-arm dumbell extension is performed in a manner that looks like William Wallace in *Braveheart* pulling a sword out of a sheath on his back over the top of his head. A dumbell is lifted up behind the head and then extended straight up. The key to successfully directing the workload to the triceps is to keep the upper arm straight, the elbow pointed toward the stars. For the best triceps tension, lift at a slight tilt of the upper body. A slow pace is especially effective with this exercise. It can be performed standing or seated. You're best to brace your body by grabbing some solid object with your free hand.

Some lifters like to use a variation of the move where a dumbell is held by both hands centered behind the head. The dumbell is then pressed straight overhead using both arms. Lou Ferrigno has frequently used this style of triceps extension.

The standard standing French press is an extension movement using a barbell or oval-

**A slow pace is especially effective for the one-arm dumbell extension.**

shaped bar with hand bars in the center. The advantage of the French press is that quite a bit of weight can be used to give the triceps a heavy load. A good workout can be attained by mixing the two-arm French press with the more concentrated one-arm dumbell extension. Warm the elbows well before doing any extensions.

**Mixed Extension Workout**

| | | |
|---|---|---|
| Standing French presses | 4 sets | 10 reps |
| Seated dumbell one-arm extensions | 4 sets | 10 reps |

Although this workout is fairly brief, it can provide a super burn in the triceps and stimulate good growth. The *one-arm dumbell extension* is also a good follow-up exercise to other heavy weight work:

| | | |
|---|---|---|
| Close-grip bench presses | 3 sets | 10 reps |
| Weighted dips | 4 sets | 10-12 reps |
| Seated one-arm dumbell extensions | 3 sets | 8 reps |

**The long rope pull works the low end of the triceps area strongly.**

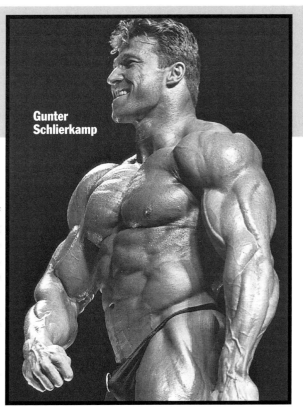

Gunter Schlierkamp

## Rope Pulls

The pushup is not the only exercise that works the low end of the triceps. Another movement also brings this specific area into play – the long rope pull. This exercise was a favorite of the late Vince Gironda, who even made a special bench to facilitate the move. To perform the exercise grasp a rope (attached to a weight pulley) and lean forward. You can support your arms on a flat bench (with knees on the floor) or perform the movement standing up, bending forward at the waist. Start with both hands behind the neck (a fairly long rope or nylon strap attachment is necessary). Pull forward, keeping the elbows down tight and make sure to get a full, hard contraction of the triceps at the end of the movement. The great stretch achieved will help you hit your lower-end triceps area with a strong enough effect to bulk up that part of the triceps very nicely.

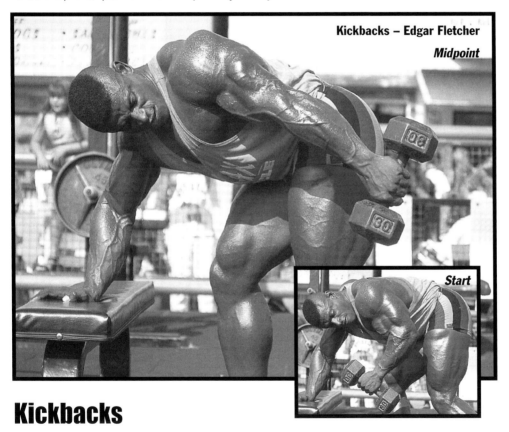

Kickbacks – Edgar Fletcher

*Midpoint*

*Start*

# Kickbacks

If you need to bring the upper area of your triceps out more evidently, the kickback exercise is the tool you will want to use to get the job done. One of the most basic and popular varieties is the dumbell kickback. Take a nice deep bend at the waist, bringing the back just above parallel with the floor, and a slight bend at the knee.

**Zero in on upper triceps development with any of a variety of kickback options.**

**The cable strap reverse-grip extension allows for a super strong triceps contraction.**

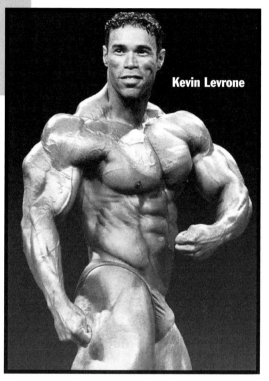

Kevin Levrone

Then take the dumbells from your shoulder area and drive them back and upward until they are roughly parallel with the flat upper body. Hold and tighten for a second, then slowly lower and repeat.

The kickback can also be done one arm at a time. A great alternative is the cable kickback, due to the high sustaining stress levels on the rear area of the upper arm throughout the movement. The cable kickback is also a great finishing exercise for a red-hot pump at the end of a full routine.

## Super Strap

Here's an exercise that will really blow away the triceps, utilizing the cable strap with a medium cable pulley and an incline bench. This move is performed with a reverse grip and the strap is attached to a pulley at about waist height. From a seated position on the bench, you start by pushing the strap almost straight out with just a slight upward angle (instead of the steep upward angle when the low pulley position is used). Contract the arms hard at the midpoint, then return under full control to the starting position.

The reverse hand grip will help work all three heads of the triceps. Position the bench so that the weights never fully touch back down until the set is over to bring about constant tension on the triceps. Make it a point to get a good strong lock-out (full and hard contraction) at the outer end of the movement for each and every rep, and a very deep, straight stretch at the return position. Focus on this action even in the latter part of the set when the pain builds up.

The triceps are a key muscle in building a strong and powerful body, and this is the key muscle to target if you want hot arms. Triceps-training is the *cornerstone* of the *prime beef* approach to building better arms – so give it top priority and the very best of your arm-training output.

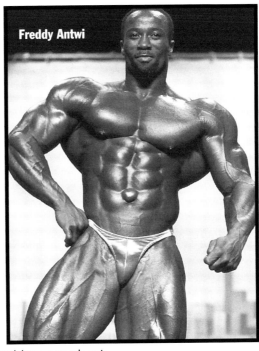

Freddy Antwi

### "Freaky" Triceps Routine – Freddie Antwi's Off-Season Workout

Triceps pushdowns:
   1 warmup set
   1 set of 6-8 reps with maximum weight
   2 sets of 8-10 reps
   2 sets of 10-12 reps
Reverse pushdowns:
   3 sets of 8-10 reps
One-arm dumbell extensions:
   3 sets of 8-10 reps
One-arm cable pushdowns:
   3 sets of 12-15 repetitions
This routine is performed following your biceps workout.

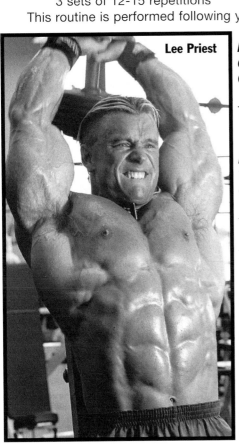

Lee Priest

### Powerlifting Champ Chris Confessore on Power Triceps-Training

Close-grip bench presses:
   "A must for triceps power."
Triceps pushdowns:
   "Develop lockout power."

### Bob Kennedy's Suggested Triceps Power Routine

Close-grip bench presses:
   3 sets of 6-8 reps
Triceps extensions:
   3 sets of 6-8 reps
Triceps pushdowns:
   3 sets of 6-8 reps

### Lee Priest on Arm-Training

"Take each set to absolute failure. If possible, cheat out a few reps and have a training partner help you with 1 or 2 extra forced reps. Don't exhaust your muscles by doing too many warmup sets or going to absolute failure on the first couple of working sets. Save your strength and energy for the final, heaviest sets."

***Richard Farley's Triceps-Training (as noted in* Max Sports & Fitness)**
Standing lat-bar pressdowns/triceps cable pressdowns
Lying triceps extensions
One-arm standing triceps pressdowns
Rope pressdowns
Close-grip bench presses with EZ-curl bar

"I go heavy virtually all the time because the triceps have three heads, and to get them all pumped takes variety and considerable work," says Richard. "It's a feeling for me. I always do 4 or 5 sets of each exercise – more than most people, but I want the work – and as long as you're eating correctly and using it you're okay. If I underate this could be considered overtraining. My reps are always between 12 and 15 for triceps."

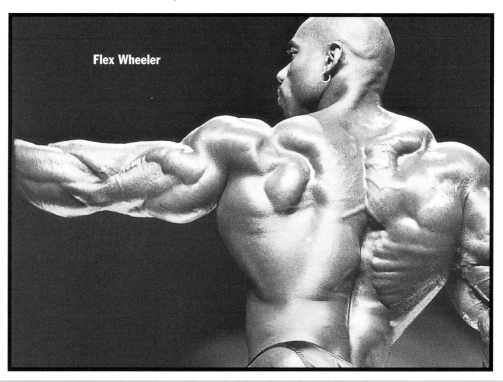

Flex Wheeler

**Be willing to experiment with your hand grip for any of the triceps movements to find the ultimate stimulation of the upper arms.**

Aaron Maddron

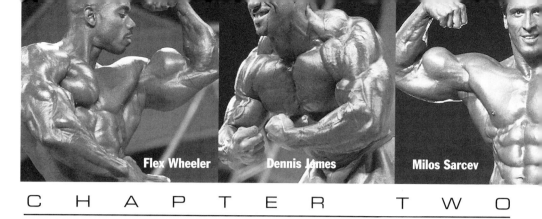
Flex Wheeler    Dennis James    Milos Sarcev

## C H A P T E R  T W O

Okay, the mandatory pep talk on triceps-training has been given. And you are now well aware of the importance of the triceps in the size of the arm. If you want big arms, build big triceps – it's almost that simple. Now on to the fun stuff, *the biceps*. Virtually no guy has to be encouraged to work his biceps. You may have to be pushed to work the tough muscle groups like legs or back, but not biceps. For some reason bigger biceps seems to be a "holy grail" for men, the one training

# Biceps Routines

pursuit that outranks all others – a pursuit that is kept alive even when good size is attained. And much of this pursuit is largely intuitive. The key to success lies in getting all of that intense interest headed down the right path. This chapter of *Arm-a-Gettin'* will help you navigate by providing some interesting information on exercises and combinations to get your biceps muscles growing bigger, broader and beefed out!

## Pressure Point

One of the central aspects of biceps-training is the correct placement of pressure during the specific exercise. This action centers primarily around the curl movement. The goal is not to see how much weight you can curl; the goal is to let the weight build up the biceps. There can be a huge difference. Many guys get into the bad habit of throwing the weight up with a boost from the hips. That isn't effective curling. Effective curling involves placing all of the pressure of the lift onto the biceps.

The first hurdle to clear in building bigger biceps is that of curling strictly. You must take the time to learn the proper mechanics of this move. A good curl makes the biceps the prime mover. The necessary technique lies in keeping the upper arm as tight against the body as possible.

**The pursuit of bigger and better biceps, the "holy grail" of bodybuilding.**

Most novice lifters will make the mistake of letting the arm travel outward as the weight goes up – a major error that can negate 20 to 35 percent of the effectiveness of the curl. Many guys keep on doing this for years – just watch them in the gym. To make it even worse, they assist the motion by involving the hips with a little boost at the bottom. This mistake also

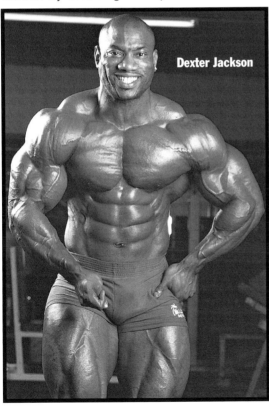

Dexter Jackson

subtracts from the effectiveness of the curl by as much as another 25 to 35 percent. Add up all that cheating and it is no wonder why some guys "curl" fairly heavy weight and have no biceps to show for it. Avoid this error if you want maximum biceps size.

Learn to put all the pressure of the repetition on the full biceps area, and nowhere else. No moving the elbows forward to get the weight up more easily. No bump from the hip to start the weight on its upward arc. Instead, just stand there and curl the weight with the power of your arms only. Proper form takes some practice to perfect, but it is worth the time. Once you get it right your arms should take off. Maybe the main reason you currently do not have a large pair of biceps is simple – they aren't receiving *the full amount of pressure* they should be during the curl motion.

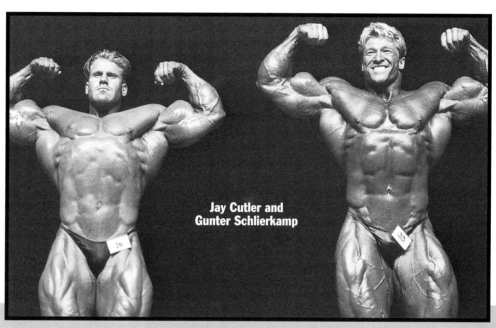

Jay Cutler and
Gunter Schlierkamp

## Improper form can take away as much as 50 percent of the effectiveness of your curling.

Curling in the correct manner may initially cause your poundages to drop. However, more direct pressure will be applied to your arms. For instance, if you are now curling 100 pounds but only at 50 percent effectiveness (due to the use of the hips and elbows drifting forward during the curl), your biceps are receiving only a 50-pound stimulation. A curl of just 70 pounds would be technically lighter but if performed correctly it would give the biceps an additional 20 pounds of overall stimulation. This factor is multiplied by the full set and full group of sets in your biceps routine for an overall weight range to show the total training effect on the biceps. If you were performing 10 repetitions per set for 4 sets, here is how it breaks down when comparing assisted vs. non-assisted curling:

## Cheat Curling

| WEIGHT | EFFICIENCY | REPS | SET | TOTAL EFFECT |
| --- | --- | --- | --- | --- |
| 100 pounds | 50% | 10 | 1 | 50 x 10 = 500 pounds |
| 100 pounds | 50% | 10 | 1 | 50 x 10 = 500 pounds |
| 100 pounds | 50% | 10 | 1 | 50 x 10 = 500 pounds |
| 100 pounds | 50% | 10 | 1 | 50 x 10 = 500 pounds |

The overall effect of the cheat curling for 4 sets of 10 repetitions with 100 pounds at 50 percent efficiency would be a weight load of 2000 pounds total on the biceps. Compare that with using only 70 pounds but curling the weight in the proper manner with total effectiveness:

# Strict Curling

| WEIGHT | EFFICIENCY | REPS | SET | TOTAL EFFECT |
|---|---|---|---|---|
| 70 pounds | 100% | 10 | 1 | 70 x 10 = 700 pounds |
| 70 pounds | 100% | 10 | 1 | 70 x 10 = 700 pounds |
| 70 pounds | 100% | 10 | 1 | 70 x 10 = 700 pounds |
| 70 pounds | 100% | 10 | 1 | 70 x 10 = 700 pounds |

The overall effect of strict curling 70 pounds at 100 percent efficiency for 4 sets of 10 reps would put *2800 pounds total resistance on the biceps.* Even though lighter weight was used, more overall resistance was placed directly on the target area, the biceps. That's why strict curling builds bigger biceps.

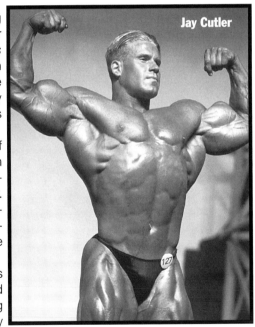
Jay Cutler

Strict curling also has the benefit of a wider range of motion (ROM) than does improper curling, as well as lighting up the neural pathways much better. Strict curling, putting the proper pressure on the biceps, is essential for maximum arm development and noticeable muscle gains.

Now consider the effect of time, as you slowly build up to a strict 100-pound curl. You can do that by first mastering the 70-pound curl in strict fashion. Only then should you move up to 75 pounds, 80 and so forth, until you are strict curling what you formerly had to cheat to get up. But using the strict approach the effect on the biceps is substantial – and they will gain substantially.

**Strict curling works the biceps muscles through a wider range of motion than does improper curling.**

**Strict Curling**

| WEIGHT | EFFICIENCY | REPS | SET | TOTAL EFFECT |
|---|---|---|---|---|
| 100 pounds | 100% | 10 | 1 | 100 x 10 = 1000 pounds |
| 100 pounds | 100% | 10 | 1 | 100 x 10 = 1000 pounds |
| 100 pounds | 100% | 10 | 1 | 100 x 10 = 1000 pounds |
| 100 pounds | 100% | 10 | 1 | 100 x 10 = 1000 pounds |

Now the overall effect is even more dramatic. The total training adds up to *4000 pounds of pressure* put on the arms during the session, compared to only 2000 from the cheat-curling approach. It takes a little longer to get there but the end result is a much heavier workload actually brought to bear on the biceps. Learn the proper way to curl and watch your biceps start to stretch the tape measure more and more.

Once you learn the proper way to perform curls, in a strict manner so as to fully effect the biceps, you are ready to put that knowledge into action for some strong gains in the size of your biceps. You are ready for *Arm-a-Gettin'* workouts.

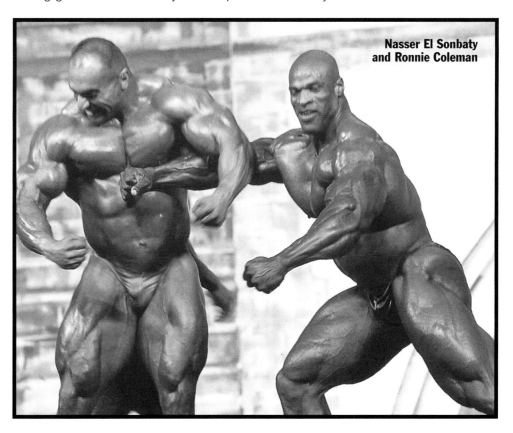

Nasser El Sonbaty and Ronnie Coleman

# Alternate Dumbell Incline Curls

The alternate dumbell incline curl is a great tool to start with in moving up to a new level of arm development. This exercise was a favorite of the legendary *Steve Reeves,* who built a fabulous pair of arms with it. Best performed on an incline bench, this move contains several beneficial elements. It allows for total concentration on the biceps – one arm at a time. It

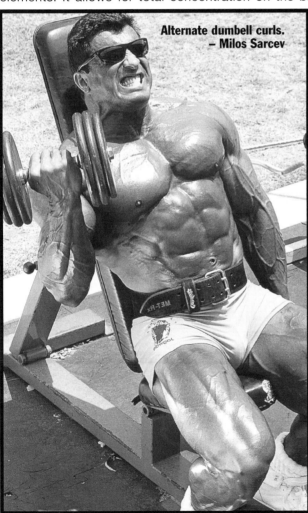

Alternate dumbell curls.
– Milos Sarcev

allows for a much deeper stretch than upright curling (the upper body is angled back, giving a longer arc to the path of the dumbell), and the wrists can be twisted as the weight comes upward, evoking even more biceps involvement. Overall it is a superb exercise that can jazz up your biceps-training.

Start the move off with your back firmly planted against the inclined bench, the dumbells down by the floor, palms facing inward. Curl one weight upward, leaving the other hanging. As the dumbell comes up, slowly rotate the wrist so that the palm of the hand faces upward instead of inward. And don't stop at an even plane, bring the lower finger (pinkie) slightly higher than the lead finger. Contract the biceps hard at the top of the move, then lower the dumbell slowly, twisting the wrist back to the starting position.

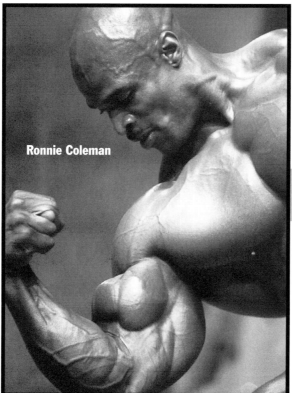

Ronnie Coleman

Take care to lower the weight slowly. Fast descent is an error that many beginners make, and a bad habit to pick up. Your biceps-training is not a sprint! Further, dropping the weight down hard and fast can tear your biceps muscle in a very nasty way. The biceps are vulnerable at this point and a slow pace is

## Biceps-training is not a sprint!

the best groove to get into. Additionally, the slower descent also keeps the biceps under better tension for a longer period of time.

Alternate the repetitions for each arm and watch as a very nice pump builds into the biceps. Keep your concentration level high, particularly in the latter stage of the rep. Generally a couple of sets of this challenging move will really get the arms going. Or you can dedicate the entire workout to just this movement. Here is how that type of routine would look:

Alternate dumbell incline curls – 4 sets x 8-10 reps

*Just 4 sets?* Yes. If you move the weights slowly and use fairly heavy poundages, 4 sets will give you a burn to the bone. Try it and see.

## Racking Out

Another prime tool for an awesome biceps pump is the use of the rack, the apparatus holding the dumbells and barbells. No, you don't lift the rack, but you do lift many of the weights from the rack. A dumbell rack workout starts with a lighter weight, perhaps 20 pounds, and performing 10 repetitions of curls. You then pick up the next heavier weight from the rack, the 25, perform 10 repetitions, and move on to the 30-pound weight, and so on up the rack. Your arms will start to give out (40 pounds, 45, 50?) and you won't be able to get in the 10 repetitions. At this point drop back down to the 20-pound weight and curl it for 8 reps. Move up again to the 25, the 30, and so on until you cannot perform the 8 reps. Drop once again to the 20-pounder. This time perform them for just 6 repetitions. Do the same up the rack again, going as far as you can. When you can no longer perform the 6 repetitions, you are finished with the biceps … which will be on fire.

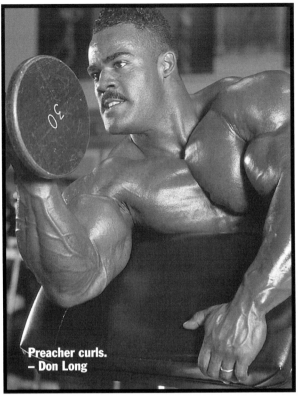

Preacher curls.
– Don Long

Dumbell curls – progressively heavier weights, sets of 10, 8, and 6 reps

## Steep Preacher Curls

The importance of a good strict curl has been stated and there is no better tool to ensure *purity of motion* than the preacher curl. The preacher bench eliminates the forward drift of the elbows as well as any assistance from the hips, making sure the only muscle lifting the weight is the biceps.

As good as the preacher curl is, it can be improved upon even more by choosing to use a preacher bench with a steep vertical angle – *the steeper the better.* Why? A steeper bench keeps the biceps under the workload longer. A steeper bench allows for a greater working range of motion. With the regular preacher bench the angle is sloped such that the arms can get a rest at the top of the lift. To circumvent this problem you have to stop short of reaching the top, resulting in a much shorter range of motion. Instead of having to take this step, switch to the steeper angle. You'll get the benefits of the full range of motion, with a deeper stretch and pressure on the arms throughout a longer range – which promotes a wider power range, bigger muscles, and more athletic arms.

> The steep preacher curl allows for a wider working range of motion for the biceps.

**A steep preacher bench allows the biceps no rest at all.**

The preacher bench can be the key component to any arm routine and the arms will readily respond. Here is a workout that employs the preacher bench with the alternate dumbell incline curl:

| | | |
|---|---|---|
| Preacher curls (strict) | 3-4 sets | 6-10 reps |
| Alternate dumbell incline curls | 3-4 sets | 6-10 reps |

## Fat Bar

Have you ever used a fat bar? Better question, *what is a fat bar?* A fat bar is a specially designed weight bar that has a thick handle area. The fat bar is as thick as the ends of the Olympic bar – but not just at the ends. It is that thick all the way through. Why concern yourself with the fat bar? The fat bar provides a unique grip on the bar that promotes a better squeeze in the biceps region. The grip is also better and conducive to a strong power surge. Once you try one of these bars you'll realize how cramped the hold on a standard skinny bar is. The fat bar can be used for standard curls or preacher curls, with which it is quite effective. Here is a routine that utilizes the fat bar:

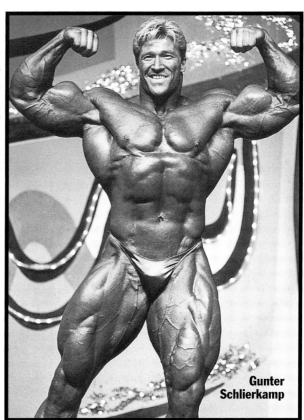
**Gunter Schlierkamp**

| | | |
|---|---|---|
| Rack out with dumbells | twice through | 8-10 reps |
| Fat-bar curls | 3-4 sets | 6-10 reps |

**Try a fat bar for your curls – you may never return to the skinny style bar again.**

# Barbell Curls

The barbell curl is the staple of most men's workout routines and should continue to be used throughout the lifetime of your training. No, you don't have to include it in every biceps-training routine or workout cycle, but it is a good exercise to have in your back pocket, ready to pop into the rotation. *Why?* This exercise promotes good gains because it squarely plants a strong workload on the biceps muscles. However, many people run dry on it because they overutilize the barbell curl, going with it all

**Don't overuse the standard barbell curl – cycle it in and out of your training over a period of time.**

the time. If you take some time away from the regular barbell curl and then come back to it later down the road, you will enjoy a nice spurt of new growth.

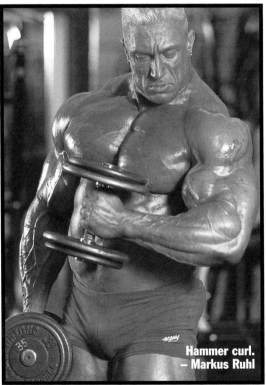

Hammer curl.
– Markus Ruhl

## Attack the Brach

Quick, *what's a brach?* The brachialis muscle is not the same muscle as the biceps muscle but is the closest arranged muscle to it in the body. The brachialis lies to the side and underneath the biceps muscles and descends down into the lower arm as well. The brachialis is an important muscle group in the scheme of things, as it lifts the biceps up, literally, when developed.

Big brachialis muscles translates into a larger arm measurement, and a pair of biceps that not only look bigger but also look much more rugged and ripped due to the unique presentation of this muscle.

The brachialis muscle is worked in a similar training arc as the biceps, but with a different slant – the hand position is changed to bring the brachialis into play. Instead of a palms-up hand position, the brachialis comes out to play when the

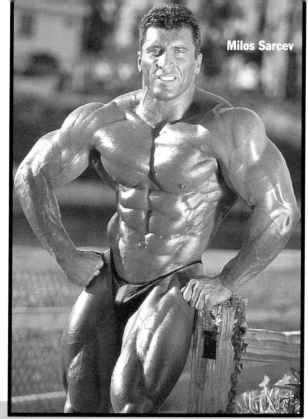

Milos Sarcev

**Want a bigger arm measurement? Work the brachialis hard and consistently and watch what happens.**

wrists face down or toward each other. Exercises they respond to are the hammer curl and reverse curl, and variations thereof. For instance, one variation, the preacher reverse curl, is absolutely tremendous for targeting the brachialis in a very strict manner.

Need more incentive for incorporating brachialis-training as part of your biceps routine? Consider this: When bulked up, the brachialis will help fill in the gap between the biceps and the forearm. Building up the brachialis will make the forearm bigger and thicker, and it will also push up the biceps (which lies over it) to a more raised position. The overall effect is terrific and makes the upper arm much fuller.

Learn this. If you want awesome arms, you have to "attack the brach" *frequently.* You won't achieve total arm development and full size unless you put in some time challenging the brachialis on a consistent basis. Here is a workout that features a couple of the better brachialis movements.

| | | |
|---|---|---|
| Hammer dumbell curls | 3-4 sets | 8-10 reps |
| Reverse-grip preacher curls | 3-4 sets | 8-12 reps |

# Top Gun Routine

Here is a great biceps workout that features several of the best biceps exercises, as well as some brachialis work:

| | | |
|---|---|---|
| Alternate (incline) dumbell curls | 3 sets | 8-10 reps |
| Strict preacher curls | 3-4 sets | 8-10 reps |
| Fat-bar reverse-grip curls | 2-3 sets | 10-12 reps |

This routine allows for super concentration and a tremendous pump of the biceps/brachialis. Start with the alternate dumbell curl on an incline bench to get you into the right frame of mind to focus intensely on the biceps. Follow the dumbell curls with strict preacher curls with the use of a steep vertical bench. Go as heavy as you can in good form, and do not rest much (1 to 1.5 minutes) between sets. Perform 3 or 4 sets to bring the biceps to a point of fatigue. Shake your arms out a couple of times and then finish them off with fat-bar reverse curls. Make sure to keep your elbows tight against your body throughout the full range of motion for the reverse curl so you have no assistance from forward elbow drift.

**The brachialis is a good filler for the gap between the upper and lower arm.**

## Burnout Workout

Need a quick burnout workout? Are there days when you simply don't have enough time for a routine but still want to keep the biceps growing? Since the biceps are an extremity of the body, their size can drop off quicker when training is withheld than with the bigger torso muscle groups (and legs). You're best to design a special routine you can switch to in the event of lack of time. You need something fast and furious that will stoke the biceps fires to burning hot – quickly! Here it is:

EZ-bar curls – 1 warmup set
EZ-bar curls – 3-4 sets x 10 reps

EZ-bar curls.
– Victor Martinez

This burnout routine is nice and compact and puts some stress on the brachialis as well as the biceps (hand position on EZ-curl bar is *angled* vs. straight). Even though you are in a hurry, get in the warmup set to make sure the elbows are ready for the move. Then load up the bar and go for it. Don't be shy about adding weight each set. You can also use the EZ-curl with a preacher bench for good effect.

**The angle of the EZ-curl bar makes it very conducive to arm growth, working both the biceps and the brachialis.**

# Concentration Curl

Are you failing to get a good pump in your biceps? Lack of a pump can be a problem as it is the almighty pump that promotes more size (along with the amount of weight lifted). Some trainers have never achieved a pump. One exercise that can restore a powerful pump to your biceps or provide you with your first pump is the concentration curl. Place this move at the end of the work-

out as a great finish to your biceps routine. The concentration curl is performed with a dumbell, one arm at a time for maximum isolation and focus. Using a dumbell in this case also allows you to rotate the wrist as the weight is raised and lowered for even more biceps involvement.

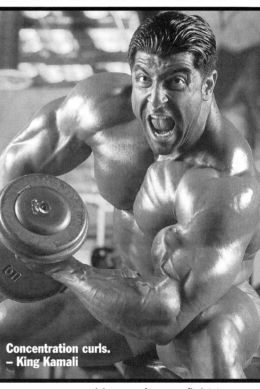

Concentration curls.
– King Kamali

To perform the concentration curl, sit on a bench with a dumbell on the floor between your legs, feet angled out for a strong bracing effect.

Grasp the dumbell and slowly curl it up toward your shoulder, contract the biceps tightly at the top, and then lower the dumbell back down. Keep the dumbell off the floor as this allows for constant tension on the biceps. Let the weight hang about 2 inches off the floor. Repeat. Don't bounce the weight at the bottom; simply lower it.

Some guys like to prop an elbow against the knee when performing this move, others let the elbow go unbraced. Use whichever approach keeps the most pressure on your biceps. As you fight to get in the final few reps, concentrate on maintaining good form and making the biceps do all the lifting. When your biceps finally give out and you cannot get it up, reach over with your free hand and assist the weight in coming up. Apply just enough pressure to get the weight up and no more. Perform a couple of these assisted repetitions, then proceed to the other arm. The concentration curl is a good exercise to employ when you find you need more pump and focus in your biceps-training.

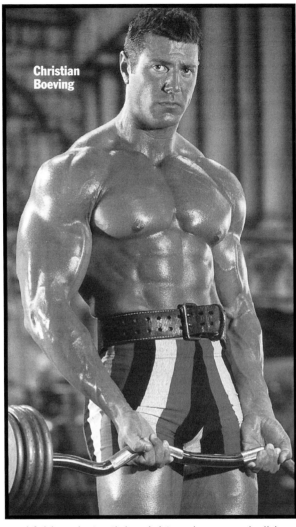

Christian Boeving

## Heavy Curls

When your concentration is just fine, you will want to work on the *monster exercise* for the biceps – the heavy barbell curl. Heavy curling is a good mass stimulator. The mind is just as important as the body in the performance of the heavy curl. You simply *must* get into the mindset that you can curl some heavy iron – and then deliberately go after it. However, don't do so immediately. You'll only fail and become discouraged. Move up in a step-by-step training approach. Continue to add weight as frequently as you can.

For the heavy curl, keep the repetition range between 6 and 8. Once you can put up 8 good reps, increase the weight again. And again. Keep after the poundage. It is possible to curl fairly substantial weight and you can build your curl poundage far beyond your current capacity. Heavy curls will translate into heavy gains in the biceps, so begin to venture into the range beyond your current workload.

## Super Pump

If you are looking for another pumping exercise in addition to the concentration curl, try the steep-incline preacher curl – without going all the way up or down. Normally you want a full range of motion in your curling action. However, for a change of pace and an incredible pump, try stopping the movement before the top, as well as stopping it before reaching the full low end of the movement. This technique will help you concentrate the work to a narrower range, and make sure the biceps receive absolutely no rest at all. Perform it on the steep incline bench to guarantee the purity of the lift, and to promote a pump that will just about burn your arms up.

If you definitely want a knockout routine in just two exercises, try the heavy curl followed up with the steep-incline preacher in a narrow range.

| | | |
|---|---|---|
| Heavy curls | 3-4 sets | 6-8 reps |
| Steep-incline preacher curls (nonlock) | 3 sets | 10 reps |

## Wise Warmup

It is a good idea to warm up the elbow area before performing any curling motion, *even if you have been lifting in previous exercises.* The stretch-out action of the biceps during the curl is quite unique and needs to be performed with a non-weight-bearing load and a light weight load before you move the iron in a serious manner. The warmup is crucial to allow you longevity in your training. A painful elbow or insertion area can limit your ability to curl or even curtail it altogether, which will bring to end your biceps gains for an extended period

**For heavy curls, keep the repetition range between 6 and 8 per set.**

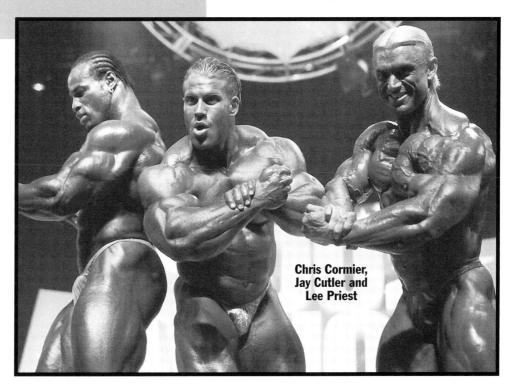

Chris Cormier,
Jay Cutler and
Lee Priest

of time. Avoid this problem by paying serious attention to a good biceps warmup, with particular focus on the elbow area and getting it ready to go. Also perform some twisting action with the wrists to prepare for any turning action in the curls you will be performing. Even if you are in a hurry, take the time to warm up.

## Cable Action

The cable is a favorite of many top bodybuilders in bringing more *sizzle* into their biceps-training. Cable training can be used as a substitute for regular barbell curls, dumbell curls, or even reverse curls. Why use a cable? As noted in the triceps section, cables supply continuous tension. Once you pick up a cable handle the tension remains on until you let go. A barbell and dumbell can be put into position where the resistance is almost nonexistent. The cable, on the other hand, keeps pulling at your muscles and forcing them to always respond. The standing cable curl, one-arm cable curl, and reverse-preacher cable curl are all top-rate exercises that can be mixed into a routine.

## Shock the Rocks!

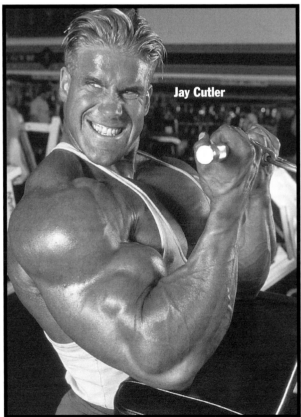

Jay Cutler

Sometimes you have to shock your biceps to get them growing again. One way to shock the rocks is to set up a workout that can be performed on a day when you have a little extra time. Begin in the morning with a session that consists of two or three biceps moves for a few sets each. Rest for an hour, then perform just a few exercises for a couple of sets. Another hour later perform one of the exercises for 2 or 3 sets. An hour later perform one of the exercises for a single set to burnout, with a weight that allows for 8 repetitions. Wait an hour and do it again.

Try to get in six to eight workouts on the biceps during the day, spaced out to about an hour apart. Then take the next few days off with extra rest and sleeping time, eat well, and watch what happens. Some guys report a noticeable spurt of growth in the biceps a few days after this shocking routine.

## Close-Grip Chins

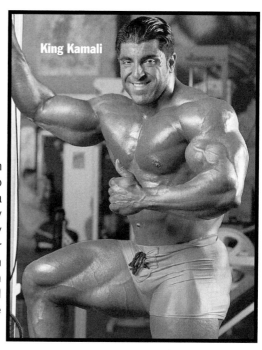

King Kamali

Tired of the same old stuff in your arm routine? Consider trying *the chinup* to work the biceps in a new way. Use a close underhand grip, and go all the way down in the bottom position, all the way up in the top. Focus on making your biceps carry the load, contracting them hard in the up position. Once you can perform double-digit repetitions, add weight to your body for more muscle stimulation.

## Take Control of your Biceps-Training

Be sure to *curl honestly* if you want your biceps to grow. *Guard against cheating.* Don't let the elbows drift forward and avoid the hip boost at all times. Add variety to your biceps workouts by trying something different than the standard biceps exercises that most trainers rep out on.

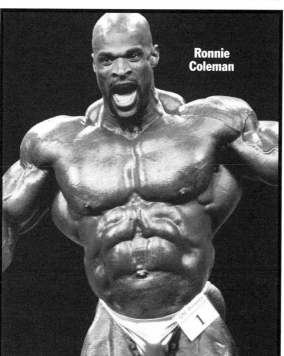

Ronnie Coleman

"Despite being a classic mass builder, the alternate dumbell curl is nearly always performed past the effective range of motion until it reaches full extension at the bottom, which is a resting point. The most effective range is full contraction at the top and just short of full extension at the bottom ... maintain tension."
– *Multi-Mr. Olympia Ronnie Coleman, on the alternate dumbell curl.*

"I use a method called *Powerbuilding.* It's a combination of powerlifting and bodybuilding. By utilizing a training partner, I can go very heavy while still maintaining proper form and tech- nique." – *King Kamali*

"Always remember, your body is a high-performance, complicated mechanism. Because you are training it to perfection with hardcore workouts it requires high-octane fuel, and lots of it." – *Aaron Maddron*

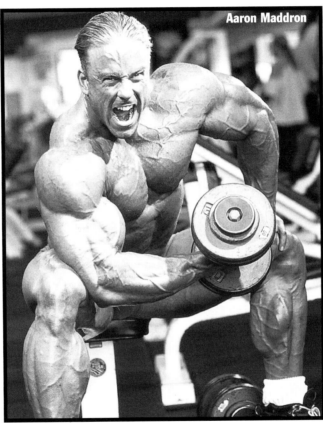

Aaron Maddron

"Working the biceps twice a week with 12 sets per session is enough for anybody." – *Ronnie Coleman*

"Do not train biceps with any other bodypart except triceps ... If you train chest with biceps, as many bodybuilders do, your chest workout depletes energy from your biceps workout."
– *Lee Priest*

"Always include preacher curls of some sort in every biceps workout. A preacher bench provides a combination of power and isolation that cannot be equaled in any other position."
– *Lee Priest*

## SOURCES

*Blood and Guts,* Yates
www.platinumphysique.com/shaundavis/main.htm
www.maxsportsmag.com/performancecondition/issue16/16pc3.htm
*MuscleMag,* September 1997
*Flex,* October 1995
*Flex,* April 2000
*Flex,* Dec. 2000
*MuscleMag, April 1998*
*MuscleMag*, December 2002

**Contributing Photographers**
Josef Adlt, Jim Amentler, Alex Ardenti, John A. Butler, Ralph DeHaan, Irvin Gelb, Robert Kennedy, Jason Mathas, Mitsuru Okabe, Rick Schaff, Art Zeller